Stages of Suicide - How to Help Your Mind

Written by:
Dr Myfanwy J. Webb

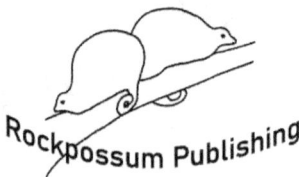

Copyright © 2023 Myfanwy J Webb

All rights reserved.

ISBN13-9780645277531

Cover design by Myfanwy J Webb

Myfanwy Webb has asserted her right under the Copyright, Designs and Patents Act 1988 to be identified as the author of this work.

This book is sold subject to the condition that is shall not, by way of trade or otherwise, be lent, resold, hired out, or otherwise circulated without the publisher's prior consent in any form of binding or cover other than that in which it is published and without a similar condition, including this condition, being imposed on the subsequent purchaser. Inquiries should be addressed to the author at myfanwy@myfanwywebb.com

myfanwywebb.com

This book is dedicated to both those who have lost and those who struggle.

Table of Contents

Preface	1
Introduction	3
Concept Explanation	4
Stages of Suicide	7
Stage 1 FALLING SHORT OF EXPECTATIONS	9
Stage 2 ATTRIBUTIONS OF SELF	13
Stage 3 HIGH SELF-AWARENESS	17
Stage 4 NEGATIVE AFFECT	21
Stage 5 COGNITIVE DECONSTRUCTION	23
Stage 6 DISINHIBITION	27
LIVE	29
References	31
Mind Monitoring Tool	33
International Suicide Hotlines	41
About the Author	46

Preface

As a researcher, I was employed to study suicides in the region where I live. I became quite passionate about trying to help keep people alive using the data from the deceased people. My aim was to turn their deaths into something useful to prevent further suicides. That way, the torment experienced by those individuals would not be in vain.

From all I read, I could not really understand what these people felt. Then I came across a structured description of what people go through and I realized that this is something that people can use to empower themselves to stop the dangerous and tragic downwards trajectory.

Introduction

This is a short explanation of the six stages of suicide with practical activities to help you to prepare for and assist your mind in the event it becomes irrational and unsafe.

Included is a mind-monitoring tool to assist you in identifying if your mind is displaying signs of reacting within the various six stages. The tool also provides actions you can do to support your mind.

At the end of this guide, you can find a list of help crisis hotlines for various countries.

Concept Explanation

Suicide as Escape from Self is a paper by Roy Baumeister, a social psychologist who described the stages that people experience prior to carrying out suicidal acts. These stages are useful indicators of whether someone is heading seriously downhill. If you understand these stages and think about times when others or yourself, have experienced these feelings, then you have a way of monitoring your internal state. Because the mind becomes increasingly incapable of thinking properly during each stage, it is worth working out what to do to help your mind before it hits that dark slope down. I'll put **Roy's words in bold italics**.

Suicide is analyzed in terms of motivations to escape from aversive self-awareness.

Therefore, a strategy to counter aversive self-awareness can help.

"As individuals habituate to the fear of self-harm and death, the desire to remain engaged with life diminishes" (Van Orden et al., 2010).

The more you can transform aversive, undesirable thoughts about yourself into favorable thoughts of self, the more you will feel free of being trapped inside an irrational and unhelpful mind.

When you are feeling good, it is worth setting aside time to prepare and work out some steps to take in preparation for bad times when you might experience indicators of pre-suicide stages. Monitoring your actions and emotions is valuable here.

A valuable first step is to identify multiple people (friends, specialist, relatives, helpline person) that you will be able to talk with, if you notice yourself highly absorbed in any of the stages and are finding it difficult to think. You can add this information into the Mind Monitoring Tool found at the end of the book. You might like to copy your information down or make a print of the tool if that helps. I have added a list of Helpline contact numbers at the end too.

In his paper, Baumeister describes the concept as:

Suicide is analyzed in terms of motivations to escape from aversive self-awareness. The causal chain begins with events that fall severely short of standards and expectations. These failures are attributed internally, which makes self-awareness painful. Awareness of the self's inadequacies generates negative affect, and the individual therefore desires to escape from self-awareness and the associated affect. The person tries to achieve a state of cognitive deconstruction (constricted temporal focus, concrete thinking, immediate or proximal goals, cognitive rigidity, and rejection of meaning), which helps prevent meaningful self-awareness and emotion. The deconstructed state brings irrationality and disinhibition, making drastic measures seem acceptable. Suicide can be seen as an ultimate step in the effort to escape from self and world.

Stages of Suicide

There are six distinct stages to prepare for:

Stage 1   Falling short of expectations

Stage 2   Attributions of self

Stage 3   High self-awareness

Stage 4   Negative affect

Stage 5   Cognitive deconstruction

Stage 6   Disinhibition

Stage 1

FALLING SHORT OF EXPECTATIONS

The causal chain begins with events that fall severely short of standards and expectations.

This is having a high standing which changes to a low standing in life or being under the pressure of too high expectations from others.

One example that comes to mind is a man I know of who had an enormous salary, was about to gain a $200k end-of-year bonus but was caught after hours, crashed out at his desk under the influence of drugs. He lost his cash bonus and his job and didn't know how to tell his wife. So, he didn't. He lost his life in his struggle.

If his mind had been operating in a rational way, he would have said to himself, *I'll look for another job...*

money is not everything...my job is not me, it isn't my identity...my wife will get over it...shit happens...such is life...maybe the next job will be better for me anyway...at least now I don't have to hide stuff anymore...I can go do drug rehabilitation etc.

Prepare your Mind

If you are at risk of having the shit hit the fan in your life, you can support yourself by having some rational responses for your mind ready for the occasion.

If you think you might fail an exam then well before your exam, you could follow through the imaginary thread of what could happen if this goes down and instead of only seeing all the negative parts, you could brainstorm all the ways you can come out of it and still be okay.

For example, *I'll have to repeat another semester, but I can find a tutor or ask that smart friend in my class if they'd give me some tips and that way, I'll still achieve my goal of passing the course... it just might take longer but so what.*

Or...*Mum and dad will explode if I don't do well, but they can't be angry forever, every single day for the rest of my life. They will calm down eventually. I'll just have to wait till they do calm down and things will get better. Then they won't expect so much of me in the future so I'll be off the hook more than I've ever been which will be way better for me.*

Another way to prepare is to imagine the worst scenario by asking the question, *What's the worst that can happen here?* Answer it with contingency plans for various scenarios that help you prepare for transforming it from dire to tolerable and then manageable. Also, there's always the potential for you to swing the pendulum fully the other way and see advantageous, bonus outcomes that sprout from something bad happening.

The Mind Monitoring Tool at the end of this book is designed to help you with preparing your mind.

For a printable PDF go to;
http://www.myfanwywebb.com/wp-content/uploads/2022/10/Mind-Monitoring-Tool.pdf

Stage 2

ATTRIBUTIONS OF SELF

These failures are attributed internally

People attributing failure internally may believe that other people are 'better than them' and may experience self-loathing. Often, they think they are different to others and feel isolated. Blame is internalized and they blame themselves rather than other people, the circumstances or things that are out of their control. (The misanthropic, always-negative people are not as at risk and are, to a degree protected, as they may not like themselves but they like others even less).

When you find yourself attributing failures internally, this may be a sign you are on that dark slope and on the way down. It may help to work out ways to attribute those failures to external factors.

If you feel that the bad stuff that happens to you is all your fault, then try drilling down and put it into a rational framework. So, for instance, you might feel crap all the time and yet your life on paper is great, so therefore you're thinking that it's all your own fault that you feel miserable. However, your misery might be stemming from external variables that happened to you in childhood such as you were constantly told how useless you were by your parents and it's hard now to accept that you are NOT useless. You weren't useless back then in the past, and you are not useless now, in the present time. You are not alone. Other men, women, adolescents, kids feel the same crappy feelings for the same reasons (and other reasons of course).

Or maybe you didn't win the job you applied for, and you assume it is your fault but maybe there was just someone more suited who also applied, or the employer already had someone in mind.

Prepare Your Mind

Reattribute failure from internal to probable external realities.

When you find yourself internalizing stuff then try to think logically and externalize it rather than internalize it. That way you are in a powerful position to work out solutions for yourself minus the detrimental self-blame. It might take some effort but after a while it may become a helpful and practical default and automatic response by your mind.

Stage 3

HIGH SELF-AWARENESS

...which makes self-awareness painful

The consequences of feeling extra self-conscious can be withdrawal from social contact including social media. People experiencing this stage have a reduced cognitive ability to empathize. It is hard for them to imagine how their loved ones would feel without them alive. Their perceptions might be largely distorted.

Some indicators that you are in this stage of the downward slope are if you start writing your posts that revolve around yourself and are devoid of others. Another sign is if you write in a detached manner about your friends and family.

A further indicator is if you feel detached and when you are surrounded by others, you feel you are in a surreal situation and that you are thinking how they have absolutely no idea what you are feeling. What may work for you is to regularly monitor your feelings and communications with these indicators in mind.

You may experience self-conscious emotions of shame, guilt, embarrassment and/or jealousy.

If you notice high painful self-awareness, then it is time to take the steps you have already worked out for yourself, such as have that specialist or friend help and support you.

Prepare your Mind

Regularly monitor your feelings and communications with people, for painful self-awareness indicators.

See if your interactions with people are lopsided. Ask yourself if you feel detached from reality during social situations.

Stage 4

NEGATIVE AFFECT

Awareness of the self's inadequacies generates negative affect...and the individual therefore desires to escape from self-awareness and the associated affect.

You feel psychological pain. You wish to escape from emotional agony. Some negative emotions you may feel are anger, disgust, guilt, fear and anxiety. The definition of negative affect in clinical psychology is one of many components of psychological distress that arise in relationship to some problematic aspect of life. It includes additional feelings such as boredom, depression, loneliness, frustration, irritability, envy, jealousy, hatred, disgust, contempt, embarrassment, self-criticism, and remorse.

This is a serious stage. A recent study found negative affectivity uniquely regulates the likelihood that interpersonal dysfunction will be accompanied by an exacerbation in suicidal ideation. Negative affectivity may reflect a tendency to turn interpersonal stress inward, biasing an individual away from external problem-solving and more toward suicidal ideas (Dombrovski & Hallquist, 2021).

Prepare your Mind

Regularly scan your emotions and rate intensity of those stemming from psychological distress. Repeat previous preparative tasks to help your mind and talk to your identified person or people for support.

Stage 5

COGNITIVE DECONSTRUCTION

The person tries to achieve a state of cognitive deconstruction (constricted temporal focus, concrete thinking, immediate or proximal goals, cognitive rigidity, and rejection of meaning), which helps prevent meaningful self-awareness and emotion.

Aspects of cognition fail to work properly. Time is perceived at an altered pace and slows down. You might look back on the preceding week and think it felt more like a month. You could, every Friday night, think back on the past week, and see if it matches up to feeling like a week. If it feels a lot longer, then this might be an indicator for you that your mind is deconstructing. It might be time for some specialist support to get yourself heading back up into that sunny light at the top of the slope.

Your concrete thinking increases. Your activities are taken over by more routine work rather than creative or contemplative activities. You are more detached about stuff. Activities can be aimed at distracting yourself.

If your mind won't let you rate yourself on this and you find it's too hard to do, try asking your friend or someone who knows you well. Or keep a diary or a on a piece of paper or notes on your phone, record the proportion of time you are being creative, doing routine stuff, feeling detached, what you are detached about and what makes you grounded, so you get a handle on what is normal for you and what isn't.

Preferably, start this data collection when you are feeling good so you have a gauge of how far you may later get from what is normal for you.

Prepare your Mind

Rate how much time you spend doing creative verses routine activities and time feeling detached verses grounded.

In this stage, your mind becomes completely absorbed in yourself and your empathy for others reduces even further. At this point it is beyond your comprehension to imagine how your family and friends would feel if they lost you.

Stage 6

DISINHIBITION

The deconstructed state brings irrationality and disinhibition, making drastic measures seem acceptable.

Meaningful thought is impaired. Thoughts become binary, black and white, yes/ no affairs.

There is behavioural disinhibition, a reduced fear of death and an increase in physical pain tolerance. You might not care what you say or do anymore. You may become more socially passive than usual, rather than dominant. Your deconstructed state may allow you to visualize dying in the absolutely irrational way of being okay with it.

High disinhibition clears the way for suicidal ideation to be enacted (Allen et al 2022). Disinhibition is characterized by lack of planning, forethought, and/or persistence. This stage is unlike negative affect as negative affect is associated with low mood, anxiety, and/or depressive cognitions (e.g., feeling hopeless/worthless). In the framework of the big five personality traits, it represents low levels of conscientiousness. When disinhibited, it is difficult to plan ahead, think things through before acting, and to persevere in the midst of distracting impulses.

Prepare your mind

Interrogate your mind as fully as you can. Look inside yourself from an outsider's point of view. Are your thoughts limited to binary conclusions? Are people telling you that you are being irrational? Are you irrational?

LIVE

As you come to recognize these signs in yourself and have practical actions planned ready for when you see these signs, then you have powerful tools to turn your mind back up to the top of the hill.

Thus, when experiencing the rational compared to the irrational state, you can see how your actions change. You then achieve an understanding of how your irrational mind attempts to wreck your thoughts.

You have the power to circumvent the process before and during all stages. The more practice you have at this, the more adept you become each time at maintaining a rational mind that helps and supports you.

> The more you understand how your thoughts and emotions respond in irrational ways the more you can transform your actions beyond the influence of an unhelpful mind to that of a supportive mind and live freely and fully.

References

Allen TA, Hallquist MN, Wright AGC, Dombrovski AY. (2022). Negative affectivity and disinhibition as moderators of an interpersonal pathway to suicidal behavior in borderline personality disorder *Clinical Psychological Science*, Sept; 10(5), 856-868

Baumeister R. F. (1990). Suicide as escape from self. *Psychological Review,* 97(1), 90-113

Van Orden KA, Witte TK, Cukrowicz KC, Braithwaite SR, Selby EA, Joiner TE Jr. (2010). The interpersonal theory of suicide. *Psychological Review* 117(2), 575-600.

Mind Monitoring Tool

STAGES OF SUICIDE – MIND MONITORING TOOL		
PEOPLE WHO WILL HELP ME People who I will talk to if my mind needs help Services for my urgent help.	Name 1:	Phone number:
	Name 2:	Phone number:
	Helpline:	Phone number:
	Hospital Emergency Dept. Name:	Address:
	Taxi/Uber to drive me ED:	Phone number:
	Emergency Services Police/Ambulance:	Phone number:
Stage 1 *Falling short of expectations*	What happened or might happen?	What could then happen to make it tolerable?
My extra notes:	Irrational ways I think about this: 1.	Rational ways for me to now think about this: 1.

| | 2. | 2. |
| | 3. | 3. |

Stage 2	Ways I attribute this internally:	Ways I can reattribute this externally:
These 'failures' are attributed Internally	1.	1.
	2.	2.
	3.	3.
	4.	4.

Stage 3 *Self-awareness is painful*	How self-conscious do I feel? Circle 0 = not at all 5 = a great deal 0 – 1 – 2 – 3 – 4 – 5 How much am I withdrawing from social contact? Circle 0 = not at all 5 = a great deal 0 – 1 – 2 – 3 – 4 – 5 Am I feeling high levels of shame, guilt, embarrassment and/or jealousy? Circle 0 = not at all 5 = a great deal 0 – 1 – 2 – 3 – 4 – 5	Rational ways to think about feeling self-conscious: Reasons why my feelings of shame, guilt, embarrassment and/or jealousy are irrational. 1. 2. 3.

Stage 4 *Negative affect*	How intense are my emotions stemming from psychological distress? Circle 0 = low 5 = very high 0 – 1 – 2 – 3 – 4 – 5	Repeat preparative tasks above. For high ratings contact **PEOPLE WHO WILL HELP ME** as identified and listed above.
Stage 5 *Cognitive de construction*	How much did past week feel way longer or shorter than a normal week? 0 = not at all 5 = very much so 0 – 1 – 2 – 3 – 4 – 5 Do I feel less grounded than usual? 0 = not at all 5 = very much so 0 – 1 – 2 – 3 – 4 – 5 Do I feel more detached than usual? 0 = not at all 5 = very much so 0 – 1 – 2 – 3 – 4 – 5 Am I less creative than usual? 0 = not at all 5 = very much so 0 – 1 – 2 – 3 – 4 – 5 Are my tasks more routine than usual? 0 = not at all 5 = very much so 0 – 1 – 2 – 3 – 4 – 5	Repeat preparative tasks above if score more than 0s For high ratings contact **PEOPLE WHO WILL HELP ME** as identified and listed above. ◯ Draw pie chart Proportion of time I feel detached vrs attached and grounded ◯ Draw pie chart Proportion of time I am creative/non creative.

	Do I feel more mentally rigid than usual? 0 = not at all 5 = very much so 0 – 1 – 2 – 3 – 4 – 5	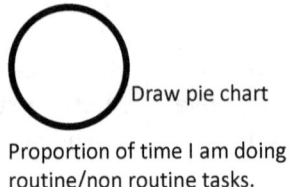 Draw pie chart Proportion of time I am doing routine/non routine tasks.

Stage 6 Dis Inhibition	How disinhibited do I feel? 0 = not at all 5 = very much so 0 – 1 – 2 – 3 – 4 – 5	Repeat preparative tasks above if score more than 0s For high ratings contact PEOPLE WHO WILL HELP ME as identified and listed above
I have left some of the pie charts blank so you can choose the content that suits you best	Am I having trouble thinking things through? 0 = not at all 5 = very much so 0 – 1 – 2 – 3 – 4 – 5	◯ Draw pie chart Proportion of time I………
	Am I having trouble planning? 0 = not at all 5 = very much so 0 – 1 – 2 – 3 – 4 – 5	◯ Draw pie chart Proportion of time I………
	Do I feel impulsive? 0 = not at all 5 = very much so 0 – 1 – 2 – 3 – 4 – 5	
	Am I having trouble persevering? 0 = not at all 5 = very much so 0 – 1 – 2 – 3 – 4 – 5	◯ Draw pie chart Proportion of time I….
	Is my thinking possibly irrational? 0 = not at all 5 = very much so 0 – 1 – 2 – 3 – 4 – 5	◯ Draw pie chart Proportion of time I….

Other measures I have worked out for myself to monitor:		

International Suicide Hotlines

Argentina
23-930-430

Armenia
2-538-194 or 2-538-197

Australia
1-800-198-313
Kids Help Line: 1-800-55-1800
Lifeline: 13-1114
Perth: (08) 9381 5555
Perth Youthline: (08) 9388 2500
Sydney: (02) 9833 2133
Launceston: (03) 6331 3355
Tasmanian callers outside Launceston: 1300 364 566

Austria
01-713-3374

Barbados
429-9999

Brazil
21-233-9191

Canada
1-833-456-4566

China
852-2382-0000

Costa Rica
506-253-5439

Cyprus
0-777-267

Denmark
70-201-201

Egypt
762-1602

Estonia
6-558-088

Finland
040-5032199

France
01-45-39-4000

Germany
0800-1110-111

Guatemala
502-254-1259

Holland
0900-0767

Honduras
504-237-3623

Hong Kong
2896-0000

Hungary
62-420-111

India
91-22-307-3451

Israel
1201 (from inside the country)
972-9-889-1333(from outside the country)

Italy

06-7045-4444

Ireland
1850-60-90-90

Japan
3-5286-9090

Lithuania
8-800-2-8888

Malaysia
03-756-8144

Mauritius
46-48-889 or 800-93-93

Mexico
525-510-2550

New Zealand
4-47-9739

Nicaragua
505-268-6171

Norway
815-33-300

Poland
52-70-000

Portugal
239-72-10-10

Russia
8-20-222-82-10

Singapore
1-800-221-4444

South Africa

0800-567-567
051-448-3000

South Korea
2-715-8600

Spain
91-459-00-50

Sri Lanka
1-692-909

St. Vincent
809-456-1044

Sweden
031-711-2400

Switzerland
143

Thailand
02-249-9977

Trinidad & Tobago
868-645-2800

Ukraine
0487-327715 / 0482 226565

United Kingdom
08457-90-90-0
ChildLine -- for children and teens
0800-1111

United States of America
988

Yugoslavia
021-623-393

Zimbawe
9-650-00 (Bulawayo)
4-726-468 0r 722-000 (Harare)
20-635-59 (Mutare)

About the Author

Dr Myfanwy J Webb worked for NSW Health researching suicide over a ten-year period investigating Mental Health, Drug and Alcohol and Coronial files. She co-authored a Submission to the Senate Affairs Reference Committee for the Inquiry into Suicide in Australia 2010. Dr Webb co-authored the Report to Coroner by Police Officer in Event of Possible Suicide 2011. She actively campaigns for implementing suicide prevention measures at sites of high risk.

She is currently a Conjoint Fellow at the University of Newcastle in the School of Medicine and Public Health.

Another book written by Myfanwy Webb is,

Wild – Life Death Encounters with Wild Animals

(Memoir Adventure) Rockpossum Publishing.

ISBN13-9780645277500

www.ingramcontent.com/pod-product-compliance
Lightning Source LLC
Chambersburg PA
CBHW072339300426
44109CB00042B/1923